How to Get Harder and Stronger Erections

Comprehensive Guide to Strengthening Your Penis for Long Lasting Sexual Experience, Harder Erection and Better Sexual Experience

Cheryl Bach

How to Get Harder and Stronger Erections

©2024 by Cheryl Bach

All rights reserved. No part of this publication may be reproduced, distributed, or transmitted in any form or by any means, including photocopying, recording, or other electronic or mechanical methods, without the prior written permission of the publisher, except in the case of brief quotations embodied in critical reviews and certain other noncommercial uses permitted by copyright law. For permission requests, write to the publisher at the address below.

Publisher: IntimateInk Press

Email: intimateinkpress@gmail.com

This book is a work of nonfiction intended for informational purposes only. The content of this book is based on the author's research, knowledge, and experience, and it is provided with the understanding that the author and publisher are not engaged in rendering legal, medical, or professional advice. The information in this book is not a substitute for professional guidance or assistance. Readers should consult with relevant professionals for advice and assistance regarding their specific situations. The author and publisher disclaim any liability for any loss or risk, personal or otherwise, which is incurred as a consequence, directly or indirectly, of the use and application of any of the contents of this book.

Cover design by IntimateInk Press

Interior layout and design by IntimateInk Press

Printed in USA

Fonts: Google fonts

Image: Freepik.com. This cover has been designed using assets from Freepik.com

For permission to use copyrighted material from this book, please contact the copyright holder listed above.

First Edition: 2024

Distributed by Amazon.com, Inc.

Cheryl Bach

Table of Contents

Introduction

In the study of human sexuality, few topics are as central, yet often overlooked, as the quality of erections. For men, the ability to achieve and maintain firm, strong erections is not just a matter of pleasure; it's a cornerstone of sexual confidence and vitality. The ability to achieve lasting erections in men plays a critical role in sexual performance and satisfaction.

Unfortunately, most men experience erection problems at some stage of their lives, which is emotionally devastating and drastically impacts their quality of life. Good erections matter because they not only play a crucial role in sexual performance and pleasure, but also overall sexual and emotional health. This book aims to provide a

How to Get Harder and Stronger Erections

comprehensive guide to improving and strengthening your penis for long-lasting, satisfying sexual experiences.

Why Good Erections Matter

Good erections are vital in maintaining sexual health, performance, and satisfaction. Men who experience low-quality erections may experience difficulties in achieving orgasm and pleasure, ultimately affecting their self-esteem and confidence. It's essential to understand that good erections are not just a matter of sexual gratification but contribute significantly to overall emotional and physical health.

Studies suggest there is a strong link between erectile dysfunction (ED) and various heart diseases such as coronary artery disease, peripheral artery disease, and hypertension. With this information, it becomes essential to prioritize your sexual health to enjoy long-lasting and healthy erections.

Importance of Sexual Health and Performance

Sexual health isn't just about not getting sick. It's about feeling good about yourself and your body, and being able to have satisfying and enjoyable sex. But sometimes things can get in the way of that, like feeling anxious or stressed, or having trouble with things like erections or finishing too quickly.

When these things happen, it's important to talk about them and get help if you need it. Because having a healthy sex life isn't just good for you, it's good for your relationships too. When you and your partner can communicate openly and enjoy sex together, it can make your relationship stronger and more satisfying.

Brief Overview of What the Book Will Cover

In this book, we're going to cover a lot of stuff to help you improve your erections and have better sex overall. We'll start by explaining how erections work, so you understand what's going on in your body. Then, we'll talk about things that can affect your erections, like diet, exercise, and stress.

We'll also go over common problems guys have with sex, like erectile dysfunction (when you can't get or keep an erection) and premature ejaculation (when you finish too quickly). And we'll give you tips and techniques for dealing with these issues so you can have more satisfying sex.

Finally, we'll talk about how important it is to communicate with your partner about sex, and how to build intimacy and connection in your relationship. Because when you and your partner can talk openly and enjoy sex together, it can make your relationship stronger and more fulfilling. So get ready to learn all about how to have better erections and better sex. It's going to be a journey, but by the end of this book, you'll have the knowledge and tools you need to improve your sex life and feel more confident and satisfied in bed.

Chapter 1

Understanding Erections

How Erections Work

Erections are the result of a complex physiological process that involves the interplay of the nervous system, vascular system, and hormonal system. When a man becomes sexually aroused, sensory signals from the brain trigger the release of neurotransmitters, such as nitric oxide, that cause the smooth muscles in the penis to relax. This relaxation allows blood to flow into the erectile tissue, filling the spongy chambers known as the corpora cavernosa and causing the penis to become erect.

Nitric oxide plays a pivotal role in the erection process by signaling the smooth muscles in the penis to relax, allowing

Cheryl Bach

blood vessels to dilate and increase blood flow. Nitric oxide is produced by endothelial cells lining the blood vessels in response to sexual stimulation, and its levels are regulated by various factors, including hormones, neurotransmitters, and physical stimuli.

Once an erection is achieved, it is maintained through a balance of continued blood flow into the penis and reduced blood flow out of the penis. This balance is controlled by the contraction of smooth muscle cells in the penis and the compression of blood vessels, which helps trap blood within the erectile tissue and sustain the erection.

Common Causes of Erection Problems

Erection problems can be caused by a variety of physical factors, including vascular issues such as atherosclerosis (hardening of the arteries), which can restrict blood flow to the penis. Other physical causes may include hormonal imbalances, neurological disorders, anatomical abnormalities, and certain medical conditions such as diabetes, hypertension, or obesity.

Psychological factors can also contribute to erection problems, particularly in cases of performance anxiety, stress, depression, or relationship issues. Negative emotions and psychological stressors can interfere with the brain's ability to signal arousal and trigger the release of neurotransmitters necessary for initiating and maintaining an erection.

Unhealthy lifestyle habits, such as smoking, excessive alcohol consumption, drug use, poor diet, lack of exercise, and inadequate sleep, can all contribute to erectile dysfunction by affecting vascular health, hormone levels, and overall well-being. Addressing these lifestyle factors is essential for optimizing erectile function and sexual performance.

Importance of Identifying Underlying Issues

Identifying the underlying causes of erection problems is essential for developing an effective treatment plan tailored to the individual needs of the patient. While oral medications like Viagra or Cialis may be suitable for some men, others may require alternative treatments such as penile injections, vacuum pumps, or penile implants to address underlying vascular or neurological issues.

Addressing underlying issues early can help prevent the progression of erectile dysfunction and reduce the risk of complications such as cardiovascular disease, diabetes, or hormonal imbalances. By treating the root cause of erection problems, men can improve their overall health and well-being and enjoy a better sexual experience.

Achieving and maintaining harder, stronger erections can significantly enhance quality of life, self-esteem, and overall satisfaction with intimate relationships. By identifying and addressing underlying issues contributing to erection problems, men can reclaim their sexual health and enjoy long-lasting sexual experiences.

In conclusion, understanding how erections work, common causes of erection problems, and the importance of identifying underlying issues are essential steps towards achieving and maintaining harder, stronger erections for a better sexual experience. By addressing physical, psychological, and lifestyle factors, men can optimize their erectile function and enjoy greater satisfaction and fulfillment in their intimate relationships.

Cheryl Bach

Chapter 2

Lifestyle Changes for Better Erections

We'll explore the pivotal role that lifestyle factors such as diet, exercise, weight management, alcohol consumption, smoking, and drug use play in determining the quality of your erections and overall sexual health. By making informed choices and adopting healthier habits, you can significantly enhance your ability to achieve and maintain harder, stronger erections for a more fulfilling sexual experience.

The Role of Diet and Exercise in Sexual Health

A balanced diet rich in fruits, vegetables, whole grains, lean proteins, and healthy fats is essential for overall health, including sexual function. Certain nutrients, such as antioxidants, vitamins (particularly vitamin D), and minerals like zinc and magnesium, play key roles in supporting erectile function and promoting blood flow to the penis.

Regular physical activity is crucial for maintaining cardiovascular health, optimizing blood flow, and enhancing erectile function. Both aerobic exercise (such as jogging, swimming, or cycling) and resistance training (weight lifting) have been shown to improve erectile function by reducing the risk of conditions like obesity, diabetes, and hypertension, which can impair blood flow to the penis.

Tips for Losing Weight and Reducing Alcohol Consumption to Improve Erections

Weight Management: Excess body weight, especially around the abdomen, is associated with an increased risk of erectile dysfunction (ED). Losing weight through a combination of healthy eating and regular exercise can improve erectile function by reducing inflammation, lowering blood pressure, and enhancing vascular health.

Moderating Alcohol Intake: While alcohol consumption in moderation may have some cardiovascular benefits, excessive drinking can have detrimental effects on sexual function. Chronic alcohol abuse can lead to hormonal imbalances, liver damage, and neurological impairment, all of which can contribute to erectile problems. Limiting alcohol intake to moderate levels (typically defined as up to one drink per day for women and up to two drinks per day for men) can help preserve erectile function.

The Effects of Smoking and Drug Use on Sexual Health

Smoking and Erectile Dysfunction: Smoking is a major risk factor for erectile dysfunction, primarily due to its detrimental effects on vascular health. Nicotine constricts blood vessels, reducing blood flow to the penis and impairing erectile function. Additionally, smoking damages the endothelial cells lining the blood vessels, further compromising vascular health. Quitting smoking is one of the most effective ways to improve erectile function and overall sexual health.

Impact of Drug Use: Recreational drug use, including illicit substances like cocaine, methamphetamine, and heroin, can have profound effects on sexual function. These drugs can disrupt hormonal balance, impair neurological function, and damage blood vessels, leading to erectile dysfunction and other sexual problems. Seeking support and treatment for drug addiction is essential for preserving sexual health and overall well-being.

By making positive lifestyle changes such as adopting a healthy diet, engaging in regular exercise, maintaining a healthy weight, moderating alcohol consumption, quitting smoking, and avoiding recreational drug use, you can significantly improve your erectile function and enhance your overall sexual health. In the next chapter, we'll explore additional natural remedies and supplements that can further support erectile health and sexual performance.

Cheryl Bach

Chapter 3

Natural Remedies for Erection Problems

There are various natural remedies for erectile dysfunction (ED) and other erection problems. From herbal supplements to dietary changes and lifestyle adjustments, these remedies offer a holistic approach to improving erectile function and enhancing sexual performance.

Common Natural Remedies for Erectile Dysfunction

L-arginine: L-arginine is an amino acid that plays a crucial role in the production of nitric oxide, a molecule that helps relax blood vessels and improve blood flow to the penis. By increasing nitric oxide levels, L-arginine supplementation may enhance erectile function. It is often combined with other supplements like Pycnogenol for improved efficacy.

Yohimbine: Yohimbine is derived from the bark of the yohimbe tree and has been used traditionally as an aphrodisiac. It works by increasing blood flow to the penis and improving nerve impulses involved in arousal. While research on its effectiveness is mixed, some men may experience improved erectile function with yohimbine supplementation.

Maca: Maca is a root vegetable native to Peru that has long been used for its purported aphrodisiac properties. It is believed to balance hormone levels, improve energy and stamina, and enhance sexual desire. While scientific evidence supporting its efficacy for erectile dysfunction is limited, some men may find maca supplementation beneficial.

Horny Goat Weed: Horny goat weed, also known as epimedium, is a traditional Chinese herbal remedy for erectile dysfunction and low libido. It contains active compounds like icariin, which may help improve erectile function by increasing blood flow to the penis and inhibiting the enzyme responsible for breaking down nitric oxide.

Ginseng: Ginseng is a popular herbal remedy used in traditional medicine to improve vitality and sexual function. Both Asian ginseng (Panax ginseng) and American ginseng (Panax quinquefolius) have been studied for their potential benefits in treating erectile dysfunction. Ginseng may improve erectile function by increasing nitric oxide production and enhancing blood flow to the penis.

Tribulus Terrestris: Tribulus terrestris is a plant extract commonly used in traditional medicine to enhance libido and sexual performance. It is believed to increase testosterone levels, which may improve erectile function and sexual desire in some men. However, research on its efficacy for treating erectile dysfunction is limited.

How to Use at Home Remedies to Increase Hardness and Duration of Erection

Pelvic Floor Exercises: Pelvic floor exercises, also known as Kegel exercises, can help strengthen the muscles involved in erectile function and improve blood flow to the pelvic area. To perform Kegels, simply contract the muscles used to stop the flow of urine for several seconds, then relax. Aim for three sets of 10 repetitions per day.

Healthy Lifestyle Habits: Adopting a healthy lifestyle can also improve erection hardness and duration. This includes maintaining a balanced diet rich in fruits, vegetables, whole grains, and lean proteins, getting regular exercise, managing stress, and getting an adequate amount of sleep each night.

Stimulating Lubricants: Using lubricants or stimulating gels during sexual activity can enhance sensation and improve erectile function. Look for products containing ingredients like L-arginine or menthol, which can increase blood flow to the penis and enhance arousal.

Mindfulness and Relaxation Techniques: Stress and anxiety can contribute to erectile dysfunction by causing muscle tension and interfering with arousal. Practicing mindfulness techniques such as deep breathing, meditation, or progressive muscle relaxation can help reduce stress and improve erectile function.

By incorporating these natural remedies and lifestyle adjustments into your daily routine, you can support erectile health and improve your sexual performance. However, it's essential to remember that individual responses may vary, and consulting with a healthcare professional is recommended before starting any new supplements or treatments for erectile dysfunction. In the next chapter, we'll explore medical interventions and advanced treatments for more severe cases of erectile dysfunction.

Chapter 4

Medical Treatment Options for Erection Problems

Various medical treatment options are available for addressing erectile dysfunction (ED), including prescription medications like Viagra and Cialis. We'll explore how these treatments work, their effectiveness, and the potential risks and side effects associated with their use.

Overview of Medical Treatments for ED

Phosphodiesterase Type 5 (PDE5) Inhibitors: PDE5 inhibitors are the most commonly prescribed medications for erectile dysfunction. They work by inhibiting the enzyme phosphodiesterase type 5, which is responsible for breaking down cyclic guanosine monophosphate (cGMP), a molecule that promotes relaxation of smooth muscle cells and increased blood flow to the penis. By blocking PDE5, these medications enhance the effects of cGMP, resulting in improved erectile function. Some of the most well-known PDE5 inhibitors include:

Viagra (Sildenafil): Viagra was the first PDE5 inhibitor to be approved for the treatment of erectile dysfunction. It is typically taken on an as-needed basis, about 30 minutes to an hour before sexual activity, and can remain effective for up to four hours.

Cialis (Tadalafil): Cialis is another PDE5 inhibitor that is approved for both on-demand and daily use. It has a longer duration of action compared to Viagra, with effects lasting up to 36 hours. This makes it a popular choice for men who prefer spontaneity in their sexual encounters.

Levitra (Vardenafil): Levitra is similar to Viagra in its mechanism of action and duration of action. It is typically taken 30 minutes to an hour before sexual activity and can remain effective for up to five hours.

Other Prescription Medications

In addition to PDE5 inhibitors, there are other prescription medications that may be used to treat erectile dysfunction, either alone or in combination with other therapies.

These include:

Alprostadil: Alprostadil is a prostaglandin E1 analogue that can be administered as an injection into the penis or as a urethral suppository. It works by dilating blood vessels and increasing blood flow to the penis, resulting in an erection.

Testosterone Replacement Therapy (TRT): Testosterone replacement therapy may be prescribed for men with low testosterone levels, which can contribute to erectile dysfunction. TRT can be administered via injections, patches, gels, or pellets.

How These Treatments Work

PDE5 inhibitors like Viagra and Cialis work by enhancing the effects of nitric oxide, a molecule that promotes relaxation of smooth muscle cells in the penis and increases blood flow. When a man is sexually stimulated, nitric oxide is released in the erectile tissue, leading to the production of cyclic guanosine monophosphate (cGMP). This molecule relaxes the smooth muscle cells in the penis, allowing blood to flow in and produce an erection.

However, in men with erectile dysfunction, the enzyme phosphodiesterase type 5 (PDE5) breaks down cGMP too quickly, leading to difficulty achieving or maintaining an erection. PDE5 inhibitors block the action of PDE5, allowing cGMP levels to remain elevated and promoting improved erectile function.

Risks and Side Effects Associated with Medication Use

While PDE5 inhibitors are generally safe and well-tolerated, they can cause certain side effects in some men. Common side effects may include headache, flushing, indigestion, nasal congestion, and dizziness. In rare cases, more serious side effects such as priapism (prolonged erection lasting more than four hours), sudden hearing loss, or vision changes may occur. It's essential to consult with a healthcare professional before starting any medication for erectile dysfunction to discuss potential risks and determine the most appropriate treatment approach.

In addition to side effects, PDE5 inhibitors may interact with certain medications or medical conditions, so it's crucial to disclose your full medical history and current medication regimen to your healthcare provider before starting treatment.

In conclusion, prescription medications like Viagra, Cialis, and others offer effective treatment options for erectile dysfunction by enhancing blood flow to the penis and promoting improved erectile function. However, they are not suitable for everyone, and it's essential to weigh the potential risks and benefits with your healthcare provider to determine the most appropriate treatment approach for your individual needs. In the next chapter, we'll explore advanced treatment options for men with more severe or refractory erectile dysfunction.

Chapter 5

Alternative Treatments for Erection Problems

There are alternative treatments for erectile dysfunction (ED) beyond medication, including penile injections, vacuum pumps, and penile implants. These alternative options offer effective solutions for men who may not respond to or prefer not to use oral medications. We'll also discuss how to determine which alternative treatment may be right for you based on your individual needs and preferences.

Overview of Alternative Treatments

Penile Injections: Penile injections involve the administration of medication directly into the shaft of the penis to induce an erection. The most commonly used medication for penile injections is alprostadil, a prostaglandin E1 analogue that works by dilating blood vessels and increasing blood flow to the penis. Penile injections are typically self-administered using a small needle, and the erection usually occurs within 5 to 20 minutes and can last up to one hour.

Vacuum Pumps: Vacuum pumps, also known as vacuum erection devices (VEDs), are non-invasive devices that use negative pressure to draw blood into the penis and produce an erection. A vacuum pump consists of a plastic cylinder that is placed over the penis, along with a manual or battery-operated pump that creates a vacuum inside the cylinder. This vacuum draws blood into the penis, causing it to become erect. A constriction ring is then placed at the base of the penis to maintain the erection.

Penile Implants: Penile implants, also known as penile prostheses, are surgical devices that are implanted into the penis to provide rigidity and support for sexual intercourse. There are two main types of penile implants: inflatable implants and malleable (or semi-rigid) implants. Inflatable implants consist of two inflatable cylinders that are implanted into the penis, along with a reservoir of fluid and a pump that is placed in the scrotum. Malleable implants consist of bendable rods that are implanted into the penis, allowing it to be manually positioned for sexual activity.

How to Determine Which Alternative Treatment May Be Right for You

The first step in determining which alternative treatment may be right for you is to consult with a healthcare provider who specializes in sexual medicine. They can evaluate your individual situation, including the severity of your erectile dysfunction, your overall health, and any underlying medical conditions or anatomical factors that may influence treatment options.

When considering alternative treatments for erectile dysfunction, it's essential to take into account your preferences, lifestyle, and comfort level with different treatment modalities. Some men may prefer the convenience and discreetness of oral medications, while others may be more comfortable with self-administered injections or non-invasive devices like vacuum pumps.

Your treatment goals and expectations will also play a role in determining which alternative treatment may be right for you. For example, if you're looking for a long-term solution that provides spontaneous erections and minimal interference with sexual activity, a penile implant may be a suitable option. However, if you prefer non-invasive treatment options and are willing to undergo periodic injections or use of a vacuum pump, these alternatives may be more appropriate.

Finally, it's essential to consider the cost and insurance coverage associated with alternative treatments for erectile dysfunction. Penile injections, vacuum pumps, and penile implants may vary in cost, and insurance coverage may vary depending on your provider and policy. Be sure to discuss these factors with your healthcare provider and insurance company to make an informed decision.

In conclusion, alternative treatments such as penile injections, vacuum pumps, and penile implants offer effective solutions for men with erectile dysfunction who may not respond to or prefer not to use oral medications. By consulting with a healthcare provider, considering your preferences and treatment goals, and assessing the cost and insurance coverage, you can determine which alternative treatment may be right for you and take steps towards achieving harder, stronger erections and a better sexual experience.

Chapter 6

Psychological Factors in Erection Problems

We'll explore the significant role that psychological factors play in erection problems, including the impact of mental health on sexual performance, tips for managing anxiety and stress to improve erections, and strategies for addressing performance anxiety and relationship issues.

The Role of Mental Health in Sexual Performance

Sexual performance is deeply intertwined with mental health and emotional well-being. Stress, anxiety, depression, and other psychological factors can all influence a man's ability to achieve and maintain an erection.

Negative thoughts, self-doubt, and performance pressure can create a vicious cycle that further exacerbates erection problems.

The brain plays a crucial role in initiating and sustaining sexual arousal by releasing neurotransmitters such as dopamine, serotonin, and norepinephrine. Imbalances in these neurotransmitters, as well as disruptions in hormone levels (such as testosterone), can affect libido, arousal, and erectile function.

Past experiences, trauma, or unresolved emotional issues can also impact sexual performance. Relationship conflicts, childhood trauma, or negative experiences related to sex can create psychological barriers that interfere with intimacy and sexual satisfaction.

Tips for Managing Anxiety and Stress to Improve Erections

Stress Reduction Techniques: Engaging in stress reduction techniques such as deep breathing, meditation, yoga, or progressive muscle relaxation can help alleviate anxiety and promote relaxation. By reducing overall stress levels, men may find it easier to achieve and maintain erections during sexual activity.

Regular Exercise: Physical activity is not only beneficial for cardiovascular health but can also help reduce stress and anxiety. Exercise releases endorphins, which are natural mood lifters, and promotes better sleep, both of which can contribute to improved sexual performance.

Healthy Lifestyle Habits: Adopting healthy lifestyle habits such as getting enough sleep, maintaining a balanced diet, limiting alcohol consumption, and avoiding recreational drugs can support overall mental health and contribute to better erectile function.

Communication and Support: Talking openly with a partner about concerns and anxieties related to sexual performance can help alleviate pressure and create a supportive environment. Seeking professional counseling or therapy may also be beneficial for addressing underlying psychological issues and improving relationship dynamics.

Addressing Performance Anxiety and Relationship Issues

Mindfulness and Present-Moment Awareness: Practicing mindfulness techniques can help men stay present and focused during sexual activity, reducing the tendency to ruminate on past experiences or worry about future performance. By cultivating awareness of sensations and emotions in the present moment, men can enhance their sexual experience and reduce performance anxiety.

Cheryl Bach

Education and Reassurance: Educating oneself about normal variations in sexual response and performance can help dispel unrealistic expectations and reduce anxiety. Understanding that occasional erection problems are common and not necessarily indicative of underlying health issues can provide reassurance and alleviate performance pressure.

Couples Therapy: For couples experiencing relationship issues or communication barriers related to sexual intimacy, couples therapy can provide a safe space to address concerns, improve communication, and strengthen emotional connection. By working together as a team, couples can overcome challenges and cultivate a more satisfying and fulfilling sexual relationship.

In conclusion, psychological factors such as stress, anxiety, and relationship issues can significantly impact a man's ability to achieve and maintain erections. By addressing these factors through stress management techniques, open communication, and professional support, men can improve their mental health and enhance their sexual performance for a more satisfying and fulfilling sexual experience.

Chapter 7

Preventing Erection Problems

The Importance of Regular Checkups and Screenings

Regular checkups with a healthcare provider are essential for monitoring overall health and identifying potential risk factors for erection problems. Routine screenings for conditions such as diabetes, hypertension, cardiovascular disease, and hormonal imbalances can help detect underlying health issues early and prevent complications that may affect erectile function.

Open communication with a healthcare provider about sexual health concerns and changes in erectile function is crucial for early detection and intervention. Men should feel comfortable discussing any changes in libido, arousal, or erectile function with their healthcare provider to receive appropriate evaluation and treatment.

In addition to physical health assessments, healthcare providers may also screen for psychological factors such as stress, anxiety, depression, or relationship issues that may contribute to erection problems. Identifying and addressing these factors early can help prevent the development or worsening of erectile dysfunction.

Lifestyle Changes and Habits for Long-Term Sexual Health

A balanced diet rich in fruits, vegetables, whole grains, lean proteins, and healthy fats is essential for supporting overall health and sexual function. Certain nutrients such as antioxidants, vitamins (particularly vitamin D), and minerals like zinc and magnesium play key roles in promoting vascular health and hormone balance, which are crucial for erectile function.

Physical activity is not only beneficial for cardiovascular health but also plays a significant role in maintaining erectile function. Engaging in regular exercise, such as aerobic activities like walking, jogging, swimming, or cycling, can improve blood flow, reduce stress, and enhance overall sexual health.

Chronic stress can negatively impact erectile function by increasing cortisol levels and constricting blood vessels. Practicing stress management techniques such as mindfulness, meditation, deep breathing exercises, or yoga can help reduce stress levels and promote relaxation, which are essential for maintaining healthy erections.

Excessive alcohol consumption and recreational drug use can impair sexual function by affecting hormone levels, nerve function, and blood flow. Limiting alcohol intake and avoiding recreational drugs can help preserve erectile function and promote overall sexual health.

How to Maintain Strong and Healthy Erections

Communication with Partner: Open communication with a partner about sexual desires, preferences, and concerns is essential for maintaining a satisfying and fulfilling sexual relationship. Discussing fantasies, trying new activities, and expressing emotional intimacy can enhance arousal and strengthen erections.

Exploring Sensual and Erotic Stimuli: Engaging in sensual and erotic activities, such as massage, foreplay, or mutual masturbation, can help enhance arousal and promote strong erections. Exploring new sensations and focusing on pleasure rather than performance can reduce anxiety and improve sexual satisfaction.

Chapter 8

Kegels, Pumps and Extenders

There are three tools commonly used to improve erectile function and enhance sexual experience: Kegel exercises, penis pumps, and penis extenders. We'll discuss how each of these methods works, their potential benefits, and considerations for incorporating them into a comprehensive approach to strengthening your penis for long-lasting sexual experiences.

Strengthening Pelvic Floor Muscles with Kegel Exercises

Kegel exercises are a form of pelvic floor muscle training that involves contracting and relaxing the muscles used to control urination and bowel movements. By strengthening these muscles, men can improve bladder control, support erectile function, and enhance sexual performance.

Kegel exercises can help strengthen the muscles involved in maintaining erections and controlling ejaculation. By increasing blood flow to the pelvic area and improving muscle tone, Kegels can enhance erectile rigidity, prolong sexual endurance, and heighten orgasmic sensations.

To perform Kegel exercises, identify the pelvic floor muscles by stopping the flow of urine midstream or tightening the muscles used to prevent passing gas. Once you've located the pelvic floor muscles, contract them for a count of three to five seconds, then relax for the same duration. Aim for three sets of 10 to 15 repetitions per day, gradually increasing intensity and duration as your muscles strengthen.

Improving Blood Flow with Penis Pumps

Penis pumps, also known as vacuum erection devices (VEDs), are non-invasive devices that use suction to draw blood into the penis, resulting in an erection. A vacuum pump consists of a cylindrical tube that is placed over the penis, along with a manual or battery-operated pump that creates a vacuum inside the tube. This vacuum draws blood into the erectile tissue, causing the penis to become erect.

Penis pumps can be used to achieve and maintain erections for sexual intercourse, particularly in men with erectile dysfunction who may not respond to oral medications or other treatments. By improving blood flow to the penis and promoting engorgement of the erectile tissue, penis pumps can enhance erectile rigidity and duration, resulting in more satisfying sexual experiences.

To use a penis pump, lubricate the base of the penis and insert it into the cylinder of the device. Create a seal by pressing the cylinder firmly against the body, then activate the pump to create a vacuum. As the vacuum draws blood into the penis, it should become erect. Once an erection is achieved, slide a constriction ring over the base of the penis to maintain the erection during sexual activity.

Enhancing Penis Size and Function with Extenders

Penis extenders, also known as penile traction devices, are devices designed to gradually stretch the penis over time, resulting in increased length and girth. These devices typically consist of a base ring, adjustable rods, and a traction mechanism that applies gentle tension to the penis, encouraging tissue expansion and growth.

Penis extenders are often used by men seeking to increase their penis size or address concerns about curvature or asymmetry. By promoting tissue expansion and cell proliferation, penis extenders can lead to permanent gains in

Chapter 9

Tantra and Other Holistic Practices for Better Erections

There are many holistic approach to improving erections example, practices like tantra, meditation, yoga, and acupuncture. These ancient techniques offer a comprehensive approach to sexual health and relationships, focusing on the mind-body connection and promoting overall well-being for harder, stronger erections and better sexual experiences.

Understanding Tantra and Its Impact on Sexual Health

Tantra is a spiritual and philosophical tradition originating from ancient India that emphasizes the integration of mind, body, and spirit to achieve heightened states of consciousness and spiritual awakening. In the context of sexuality, tantra promotes the cultivation of sexual energy (known as Kundalini) for the purpose of spiritual growth, intimacy, and connection with oneself and others.

Tantra offers a variety of practices and techniques aimed at enhancing sexual health and relationships. These may include mindfulness exercises, breathwork, meditation, sensual massage, and conscious lovemaking rituals. By fostering deep relaxation, presence, and connection with one's partner, tantra can help reduce performance anxiety, enhance arousal, and improve overall sexual satisfaction.

Tantra emphasizes the importance of cultivating sexual energy and channeling it throughout the body, which can have a positive impact on erectile function. By promoting relaxation, reducing stress, and increasing awareness of bodily sensations, tantra can help men achieve and maintain harder, stronger erections and experience more fulfilling sexual encounters.

The Benefits of Meditation on Sexual Performance

Meditation is a powerful tool for promoting mindfulness, reducing stress, and enhancing overall well-being, all of which are crucial for optimal sexual performance. By practicing meditation regularly, individuals can learn to quiet the mind, increase body awareness, and cultivate a sense of inner calm and presence, which can positively impact sexual function and satisfaction.

Chronic stress can negatively impact erectile function by increasing cortisol levels and constricting blood vessels. Meditation helps reduce stress levels by activating the body's relaxation response, lowering cortisol levels, and promoting a sense of peace and tranquility. By reducing stress, meditation can help improve blood flow to the penis and enhance erectile function.

Meditation encourages individuals to tune into their bodies and become more aware of bodily sensations, including those related to arousal and sexual pleasure. By developing greater body awareness, men can learn to recognize early signs of arousal, control ejaculation, and enhance sexual stamina and control.

Overview of Other Holistic Practices for Better Erections

Yoga: Yoga is an ancient practice that combines physical postures, breathwork, and meditation to promote health and well-being. Certain yoga poses, such as pelvic floor exercises (like the Mula Bandha), can help strengthen the pelvic floor muscles, improve blood flow to the pelvic area, and enhance erectile function.

Acupuncture: Acupuncture is a traditional Chinese medicine practice that involves inserting thin needles into specific points on the body to promote healing and balance energy flow. Some studies suggest that acupuncture may be beneficial for erectile dysfunction by improving blood flow, reducing stress, and balancing hormone levels.

Herbal Remedies and Supplements: Certain herbs and supplements, such as ginkgo biloba, horny goat weed, and L-arginine, have been traditionally used to support sexual health and improve erectile function. While scientific evidence supporting their efficacy is limited, some men may find them helpful as part of a holistic approach to sexual wellness.

In conclusion, tantra, meditation, yoga, acupuncture, and other holistic practices offer valuable tools for improving erectile function, enhancing sexual performance, and promoting overall sexual health and well-being. By incorporating these practices into a comprehensive approach to sexual wellness, men can achieve harder, stronger erections, and enjoy more fulfilling sexual experiences with their partners.

Chapter 10
Conclusion and Next Steps

As we conclude our comprehensive guide to achieving harder and stronger erections for a better sexual experience, let's recap the importance of sexual health and good erections, summarize key takeaways from the book, and offer encouragement to take action and make changes for better sexual health.

Importance of Sexual Health and Good Erections

Sexual health is an integral component of overall well-being, contributing to physical, mental, and emotional health, as well as quality of life and relationships. Good erections play a crucial role in sexual satisfaction and intimacy, allowing men to enjoy pleasurable and fulfilling sexual experiences with their partners. When erectile function is compromised, it can have a significant impact on self-esteem, confidence, and overall quality of life.

Summary of Key Takeaways

Understanding Erections: Erections are complex physiological responses involving the interplay of the nervous, vascular, and hormonal systems. Understanding how erections work and common causes of erection problems is essential for addressing and overcoming challenges in sexual function.

Lifestyle Changes: Adopting healthy lifestyle habits such as maintaining a balanced diet, regular exercise, stress management, and limiting alcohol and drug use can promote overall sexual health and improve erectile function.

Medical Treatment Options: Prescription medications, alternative treatments like penile injections and vacuum pumps, and holistic practices such as tantra, meditation, and yoga offer effective solutions for improving erectile function and enhancing sexual performance.

Prevention and Maintenance: Regular checkups, screenings, and proactive measures such as Kegel exercises, penis pumps, and penis extenders can help prevent erection problems and maintain strong and healthy erections throughout life.

Encouragement to Take Action

Now that you have gained knowledge and insights into achieving harder and stronger erections, it's time to take action and make changes for better sexual health. Whether you're experiencing occasional erection problems or seeking to enhance your sexual performance, there are steps you can take to improve your erectile function and enjoy more satisfying sexual experiences.

Consult with a Healthcare Provider: If you're experiencing persistent erection problems or have concerns about your sexual health, don't hesitate to consult with a healthcare provider who specializes in sexual medicine. They can evaluate your individual situation, recommend appropriate treatments, and provide personalized guidance and support.

Commit to Lifestyle Changes: Take proactive steps to improve your overall health and well-being by adopting healthy lifestyle habits such as eating a balanced diet, exercising regularly, managing stress, and avoiding unhealthy behaviors. These changes can have a positive impact on your sexual function and overall quality of life.

Cheryl Bach

Explore Treatment Options: Consider exploring various treatment options for erectile dysfunction, including prescription medications, alternative therapies, and holistic practices. Discuss with your healthcare provider which options may be most suitable for your individual needs and preferences.

Prioritize Sexual Health: Make sexual health a priority in your life and in your relationships. Communicate openly with your partner about your sexual desires, concerns, and needs, and work together to create a supportive and fulfilling sexual environment.

Final Thoughts

Achieving harder and stronger erections is within reach for men who are committed to their sexual health and well-being. By taking proactive steps, seeking appropriate treatment, and adopting healthy lifestyle habits, you can enhance your erectile function, improve your sexual performance, and enjoy long-lasting sexual experiences and intimacy with your partner. Remember, you have the power to take control of your sexual health and create a fulfilling and satisfying sex life.

www.ingramcontent.com/pod-product-compliance
Lightning Source LLC
Chambersburg PA
CBHW051654250726
48653CB00007B/2648